90 Osteoporosis Juice and Meal Recipe Solutions:

Make Your Bones Strong and Healthy In Less Time

By

Joe Correa CSN

COPYRIGHT

This publication is designed to provide accurate and authoritative information in regard to the subject matter covered. It is sold with the understanding that neither the author nor the publisher is engaged in rendering medical advice. If medical advice or assistance is needed, consult with a doctor. This book is considered a guide and should not be used in any way detrimental to your health. Consult with a physician before starting this nutritional plan to make sure it's right for you.

ACKNOWLEDGEMENTS

This book is dedicated to my friends and family that have had mild or serious illnesses so that you may find a solution and make the necessary changes in your life.

90 Osteoporosis Juice and Meal Recipe Solutions:

Make Your Bones Strong and Healthy In Less Time

By

Joe Correa CSN

CONTENTS

Copyright

Acknowledgements

About The Author

Introduction

90 Osteoporosis Juice and Meal Recipe Solutions: Make Your Bones Strong and Healthy In Less Time

Additional Titles from This Author

ABOUT THE AUTHOR

After years of Research, I honestly believe in the positive effects that proper nutrition can have over the body and mind. My knowledge and experience has helped me live healthier throughout the years and which I have shared with family and friends. The more you know about eating and drinking healthier, the sooner you will want to change your life and eating habits.

Nutrition is a key part in the process of being healthy and living longer so get started today. The first step is the most important and the most significant.

INTRODUCTION

90 Osteoporosis Juice and Meal Recipe Solutions: Make Your Bones Strong and Healthy In Less Time

By Joe Correa CSN

The major risk factors that lead to fragile bones are genetics and family history of osteoporosis, a poor diet with a lack of calcium and vitamin D, alcohol consumption and smoking, a history of rheumatoid arthritis, and a low body weight. When combined together, these risk factors could have devastating effects on your bones.

Fortunately, some small lifestyle changes have proven to help improve bone density and prevent osteoporosis. These changes include a healthy and balanced diet, regular and adequate exercise, calcium and vitamin D supplements, and finally avoiding alcohol and cigarettes.

Our body is a magnificent living structure with the amazing ability to regenerate and heal itself. With some small daily habits, you can actually do wonders and prevent this unfortunate disease. This book is the first step in that direction. It contains osteoporosis preventing and curing juice and meal recipes that are based on natural and healthy ingredients to help your body defend itself.

Foods that are rich in calcium include dark leafy greens and dairy foods. While there is evidence that high amounts of oxalates in vegetables such as spinach, leeks, and beets hinder calcium absorption, people who consume a balanced diet will not be affected. A diet rich in grains, seeds, whole grains and seafood contain high amounts of magnesium which is essential for calcium absorption and retention.

These juice and meal recipes are healthy, delicious, and easy to make! Try them all and see how your bones start to feel.

90 OSTEOPOROSIS JUICE AND MEAL RECIPE SOLUTIONS: MAKE YOUR BONES STRONG AND HEALTHY IN LESS TIME

MEALS

1. Three cheese pizza

A cup of cheese contains four times the amount of calcium in a cup of milk. In particular, mozzarella cheese contains a high amount of calcium. Cheese is also high in protein, contains vitamin A, B12 and other important vitamins that help increase immune system and energy levels.

Ingredients:

- 1 pack Unbaked pizza crust
- 1 Tbsp. tomato paste
- 1 cans Diced tomatoes
- ½ cup Mozzarella cheese, shredded
- ½ cup Parmesan cheese, grated
- ½ cup Romano, cheese
- 1 Tbsp. Oregano
- 1 Tbsp. Basil

- 1 Tbsp. Garlic

- 1 Tbsp. Onion

- 2 Tbsp. Olive oil

Preparation:

Preheat the oven in 400°F.

Prepare the unbaked pizza crust by spreading olive oil on top of the crust.

Over medium-heat, sauté garlic until light brown and onion until translucent. Pour canned tomatoes and add the tomato paste. Simmer over low heat. Add the herbs, salt and pepper. Stir regularly. Continue cooking over low heat until consistency of the pizza sauce thickens.

Place cheese on top of the sauce. Bake the pizza in the oven for 15 minutes.

Amount per Serving:

Serves: 5 • serving size: 229g

Calories 457

Total Fat 21.6g, Cholesterol 47mg

Sodium 1296mg, potassium 248mg

Total carbohydrates 43.5g, sugars 7.4g

Protein 23.2g

Vitamin A 27% • Vitamin C 21% • Calcium 51% • Iron 16%

2.   Buttermilk pecan cake

A great substitute for whole milk is skim milk or low-fat milk. It contains the same amount of calcium with less fat and cholesterol. Low-fat and fat-free milk is formulated to include vitamin D which helps the body absorb the calcium. Dairy products provide the body with essential nutrients for optimal bone health and development.

Ingredients:

- 1/2 cup Olive oil

- 1 1/2 cups Honey

- 3 Eggs

- 2 1/4 cups Flour

- 1 tsp. Salt

- 3 1/2 tsp. Baking powder

- 1/4 cups Low-fat milk

- 1 tsp. Vanilla extract

Pecan butter:

- 2 cups Pecans

- 1/8 tsp. Cinnamon

Preparation:

To make the pecan butter, toast the pecan on a small

roasting pan in 300 F for 5-10 minutes in the oven. Mix the pecan every now and then to avoid burning it then cool. Put in a food processor and blend until consistency becomes thick and creamy. Add the cinnamon.

Preheat oven to 350F.

Beat the olive oil and honey until fully blended. For a light and fluffy cake, increase the speed of the mixer to high for the last two minutes. In a separate bowl beat the eggs thoroughly and add into the olive oil and honey mixture. Add the flour, baking soda and salt. Beat on low speed until fully incorporated. Do not over mix to avoid a tough cake. Add the milk and vanilla and beat on low for 30 seconds. Increase the speed to high and beat for another 2 minutes.

Pour the batter into a greased 9x13 pan and bake for 25-30 minutes.

Cool at room temperature before slathering the pecan butter on top of the cake.

Amount Per Serving:

Serves: 6 • Serving size: 162 g

Calories 599

Total Fat 24.8 g, Cholesterol 123mg

Sodium 535mg, potassium 434mg

Total carbohydrates 89.3g, sugars 51.3g

Protein 9.1 g

Vitamin A 12% • Vitamin C 17% • Calcium 0% • Iron 17%

3.　　Mango banana strawberry smoothie

Yogurt is low in sugar yet packed with protein, calcium and live bacterial cultures that is essential for the immune system. One cup serving of low-fat yogurt provides a full 42% average daily calcium need.

Ingredients:

- 1 Mango, sliced

- 1 cup Strawberry

- 1 Banana, sliced

- 1 Low-fat yogurt

Preparation:

Throw in all ingredients in a blender, blend well and enjoy!

Amount Per Serving:

Serves: 1 • Serving size: 262 g

Calories 151

Total Fat .8 g, Cholesterol 0 mg

Sodium 3 mg, potassium 643 mg

Total carbohydrates 38.0 g, sugars 21.5 g

Protein 2.3 g

Vitamin A 2% • Vitamin C 158% • Calcium 3% • Iron 5%

4.   Chocolate almond milk pudding

The amount of calcium present in one cup of almond is almost equivalent to that amount of calcium present in a cup of milk. Almonds contain a high amount of dietary fiber and protein which help satisfy the appetite.

Ingredients:

- 2 1/2 cups Almond milk

- 1/2 cup Cocoa powder

- 1/2 cup Honey

- 1/8 tsp Salt

- 3 Tbsp. Cornstarch

- 1 tsp Vanilla extract

Preparation:

In a medium saucepan over medium heat, pour the almond milk, cocoa powder, honey and salt. Use a whisk to occasionally stir the mixture. Boil lightly until small bubbles appear. Do not bring to a full boil. Add the cornstarch into the simmering almond milk mixture. Mix completely until cornstarch is well blended and lumps do not appear. Continue simmering until consistency is thick. Add the vanilla extract. Stir and remove from heat.

Transfer into small serving cups and cool.

Amount Per Serving:

Serves: 4 • Serving size: 193 g

Calories 489

Total Fat37.2 g, Cholesterol 0 mg

Sodium 99 mg, potassium 666 mg

Total carbohydrates 44.8 g, sugars 30.3 g

Protein 5.4 g

Vitamin A 0% • Vitamin C 7% • Calcium 4% • Iron 23%

5.   Okra tomato soup

Okra contains high amount of fiber, folates, vitamins A, B6, C and minerals that are essential for the body. A cup of okra provides 8% of dietary serving of calcium. It is also rich in manganese that provides better calcium absorption and phosphorous.

Ingredients:

- 1 cup Okra, sliced into 3/4"
- 2 400g. canned Tomato sauce
- 1 Tbsp. Garlic
- ¾ cup Red bell pepper
- 1 Onion
- 1 Tbsp. Fresh thyme
- 1 Tbsp. Olive oil
- 3 cups Chicken broth
- Salt and pepper to taste

Preparation:

Over medium heat, sauté garlic until brown and onion until translucent. Add the green bell pepper. Pour in the cans of diced tomatoes and chicken broth. Simmer for 5 minutes. Add the okra and simmer for another 5 minutes. Add the salt and pepper to taste and garnish with fresh thyme.

<u>Amount Per Serving:</u>

Serves: 5 • Serving size: 365 g

Calories 111

Total Fat 4.1 g, Cholesterol 0 mg

Sodium 1300 mg, potassium 786 mg

Total carbohydrates 14.4 g, sugars 9.1 g

Protein 6.0 g

Vitamin A 23 % • Vitamin C 60 % • Calcium 6% • Iron 16 %

6.   Cream of broccoli soup

Among the non-dairy sources of calcium, next to dark leafy greens, broccoli is considered to be second in the amount of calcium it contains. A cup of broccoli contains more than 40 mg. of calcium. It is also an excellent source of fiber, vitamins C, B6, A, iron, phosphorous, potassium, selenium, riboflavin and other minerals which makes this vegetable a super-food.

Ingredients:

- 3 cups Broccoli
- 2 Tbsp. Onion
- ½ cup Celery, chopped
- 3 cups Chicken broth
- 1 Tbsp. Garlic
- 1 Tbsp. Olive oil
- ¼ cup Onion leeks
- 1 cup Low-fat milk
- 1/8 Tsp. Parsley
- 1/8 Tsp. Thyme
- 1 Tbsp. Bay leaf
- 1/8 tsp. Salt

- 1/8 tsp. Pepper

- ½ cup Croutons

Over medium heat, sauté onions, garlic, leeks, and celery in olive oil. Sauté until onion is translucent, garlic is slightly brown, leeks and celery barely softened. Add the broccoli then add the chicken stock. Lower heat, cover pan with a lid and cook until broccoli is soft. Remove from heat and cool. Transfer into a food processor and puree together with the herbs. Season with salt and pepper. Serve with croutons on top.

Amount Per Serving:

Serves: 4 • Serving size: 353 g

Calories 145

Total Fat 5.3g, Cholesterol 11mg

Sodium 789mg, potassium 558mg

Total carbohydrates16.1 g, sugars 5.4g

Protein 8.9g

Vitamin A 16% • Vitamin C 105% • Calcium 14% • Iron 9%

7. Cod with rosemary vinaigrette topped on green beans

Green beans are a rich source of iron, folate, riboflavin, vitamins A, C, K, magnesium and potassium. A diet rich in vitamin K is associated with lesser risk in bone fracture, improves calcium absorption and reduces urinary excretion of calcium.

Ingredients:

- 4 Cod fillets, skinless and boneless
- 2 cups Green beans, cut into 2"
- 2 Sweet onions
- 1 cup Cherry tomatoes, pierced with a fork or knife on top
- 2 Tbsp. Extra-virgin olive oil
- Salt and pepper to taste
- Rosemary vinaigrette:
- 2/3 c. extra-virgin olive oil
- 1/3 cup. Lemon juice
- 1 tsp. Lemon zest
- 1 Tbsp. Rosemary
- 1 Tbsp. Parsley

- 1 Tbsp. Garlic

- 3 tsp Dijon mustard

- 2 tsp. Honey

- ½ tsp. Black pepper

- Salt to taste

Preparation:

To prepare the vinaigrette, wash thoroughly two lemons before zesting to remove coated wax. Zest one lemon then juice both. In a small bowl, combine lemon zest, lemon juice, mustard, honey, rosemary, parsley, garlic, and black pepper. Whisk briskly. Slowly pour in the olive oil. Mix thoroughly until the consistency becomes slightly creamy. Season with salt to taste.

In a skillet, heat the olive oil over high heat. Place the cod just before smoke becomes visible. Sear for 2-3 minutes or until a golden crust on the fish comes out. Carefully flip the fish on the other side and sear for another 2-3 minutes or until fish is opaque and flaky. Remove from heat and set aside.

In the same skillet, over medium heat, sauté the onions and tomatoes, pierced on top to allow the juices to come out. Throw in the green beans and cook until tender but crisp. Transfer to a plate. Layer the cod on top, sprinkle with rosemary vinaigrette on top and enjoy!

<u>Amount Per Serving:</u>

 Serves: 4 • Serving size: 204 g

Calories 356

Total Fat34.1 g, Cholesterol 0mg

Sodium 91 mg, potassium 336mg

Total carbohydrates15.5 g, sugars 7.2g

Protein 2.4 g

Vitamin A 17 % • Vitamin C 37 % • Calcium 6% • Iron 7 %

8.   Canned sardines

Consuming fish containing its bones is another way to inject a diet rich in calcium. Canned sardines also provide the essential fatty acids such as the omega 3,6,9, and vitamin D which is needed for bone absorption

Ingredients:

- 1 bottle Spanish sardines
- 1 Tbsp. Garlic
- 250 g. Uncooked pasta

Preparation:

Boil the pasta over medium heat in water sprinkled with salt. Boil until pasta is al dente. Remove from heat and transfer to a plate.

Over medium heat, sauté garlic until brown. Throw in the content of a bottle of Spanish sardines and stir for about 2-3 minutes. Remove from heat. Transfer on top of the cooked pasta. Enjoy!

Amount Per Serving:

Serves: 2 • Serving size: 135 g

Calories 379

Total Fat 3.6 g, Cholesterol 100mg

Sodium 64mg, potassium 264mg

Total carbohydrates 69.8g, sugars 0g

Protein 15.9g

Vitamin A 1% • Vitamin C 7% • Calcium 2% • Iron 26%

9.   Stir fried chicken in collard greens

Collard greens are a good source of calcium, dietary fiber, as well as vitamins A and C. They are low in sodium and fat. Collard greens are also used to detoxify harmful body toxins.

Ingredients:

- 300 g. Chicken breast, cut into strips
- 2 Tbsp. Garlic, chopped
- 1 package Frozen and chopped collard greens
- 2 Tbsp. olive oil
- Salt and pepper to taste
- ½ cup Apple cider vinegar

Preparation:

Over medium heat, sauté the garlic and chicken in olive oil until chicken is golden brown. Add the collard greens. Cook until greens are wilted. Add the apple cider vinegar. Season with salt and pepper to taste. Simmer for 2 minutes. Remove from heat and serve on a plate.

Amount Per Serving:

Serves: 3 • Serving size: 216 g

Calories 278

Total Fat 13.3g, Cholesterol 86mg

Sodium 128 mg, potassium 306 mg

Total carbohydrates 5.6 g, sugars 0 g

Protein33.8 g

Vitamin A 40% • Vitamin C 33% • Calcium 9 % • Iron 8%

10. Baked chicken and spinach in mushroom béchamel sauce

One cup of spinach contains 300mg. of calcium along with other vitamins, minerals and nutrients. However, it is important to know that increased consumption of spinach is counteractive to the absorption of calcium due to the high amounts of oxalate it contains.

Ingredients:

- 2 Chicken breast, fillet
- 2 cups Spinach
- 1 Tbsp. Garlic, chopped
- 1 Tbsp. Onion, chopped

Béchamel sauce:

- 2 Tbsp. Olive oil
- 4 1/2 Tbsp. Flour
- 3 cups low-fat milk
- ½ cup Button mushroom, thinly sliced
- 1 tsp. salt
- 1/8 tsp. Nutmeg powder
- 1/8 tsp. Pepper

Preparation:

In a small saucepan, over low heat, pour the milk and warm. Do not boil. Remove from heat and cover.

In another saucepan over medium heat, add the olive oil then add the flour. Stir until mixture is smooth. Continue cooking for 5 minutes until it changes color from dark to gold. Do not brown. Lower the heat. Slowly pour half of the milk and whisk briskly until the mixture is slightly wet, not runny. Whisk in the remaining milk slowly. Add the mushroom. Stir for about 3 minutes or until sauce is thick and creamy. Season the béchamel sauce with nutmeg, salt and pepper.

In a large saucepan, over medium heat sauté the garlic and onion until translucent. Add the chicken and cook for 5 minutes or until light brown. Flip on the other side and cook for another 5 minutes until light brown. Throw in the spinach and cook until wilted. Transfer on a plate and pour béchamel sauce over it.

Amount Per Serving:

Serves: 4 • Serving size: 315 g

Calories 311

Total Fat 10.8 g, Cholesterol 98mg

Sodium 815 mg, potassium 629 mg

Total carbohydrates17.7 g, sugars 9.9g

Protein 35.6 g

Vitamin A 39% • Vitamin C 9% • Calcium 25% • Iron 13%

11.   Creamy shrimp artichoke pasta

Artichokes are rich in dietary fiber, magnesium, potassium, iron, vitamins A, C, B3 and B9. One large artichoke contains 7% dietary amount of calcium.

Ingredients:

- 250 g. Pasta, uncooked
- 3 cups Low-fat milk
- 3 Tbsp. Flour
- 1 cup Chicken broth
- 1 can Artichoke hearts, drained and halved
- 1 cup Cheddar cheese, grated
- ½ cup Shrimp, peeled and deveined
- Salt and pepper to taste
- 1 Tbsp. Extra virgin olive oil
- Parsley for garnish

Preparation:

Boil the pasta over medium heat in water sprinkled with salt. Boil until pasta is al dente. Remove from heat and transfer to a plate.

Over medium heat, sauté onion and shrimp until onion is translucent and shrimp is bright pink. Throw in artichoke, cook for 1-2 minutes until color is deep. Pour in the chicken broth and simmer.

In a separate bowl, whisk milk, flour, cheese and pepper. Pour mixture into pan and stir. Cook over low heat until consistency is thick. Pour over the pasta. Garnish with parsley.

Amount Per Serving:

Serves: 5 • Serving size: 297 g

Calories 333

Total Fat 10.4 g, Cholesterol 68 mg

Sodium 395 mg, potassium 473 mg

Total carbohydrates 41.4 g, sugars 8.1 g

Protein 18.5g

Vitamin A 11% • Vitamin C 5% • Calcium 36 % • Iron 14 %

12.　　Baked potato gratin with Brussel sprouts

One cup of Brussel sprout has 37 mg calcium. Brussel sprouts are rich in fiber, manganese, potassium, thiamine, vitamins A, B6 and C.

Ingredients:

- 1 cup Brussel sprouts, chopped with ends trimmed and outer leaves removed
- 3 Large potatoes, sliced thinly
- 2 cups Cheddar cheese, shredded
- 3 Tbsp. Olive oil
- 1 Tbsp. Onion, diced
- 1 tsp. Salt
- ½ tsp. Thyme
- ⅛ tsp. Pepper
- 1 Tbsp. Parsley, chopped

Preparation:

Preheat your oven to 425°F. Grease 2-quart baking dish using a cooking oil.

Evenly spread the thinly sliced potatoes on the bottom of the dish. Set aside.

In a small saucepan, over medium heat, heat the olive oil.

Add the onion, salt, pepper, thyme and coarsely chopped Brussel sprouts. Sauté until onion is translucent and Brussel sprouts' outer covering is lightly brown to black. Remove from fire and pour the Brussel sprouts mixture over the potatoes until potatoes are completely covered.

Cover the baking dish with a foil and bake for 45 minutes.

Sprinkle with cheese and parsley until potatoes and Brussel sprouts are completely covered.

Bake again, uncovered, for 15 minutes or until cheese is melted.

Amount Per Serving:

 Serves: 5 • Serving size: 297 g

Calories 405

Total Fat 22.2 g, Cholesterol 66 mg

Sodium 813 mg, potassium 1024 mg

Total carbohydrates 37.3 g, sugars 3.3g

Protein 15.7 g

Vitamin A 18% • Vitamin C 100% • Calcium 36% •

Iron 10 %

13.   Garlic mussels with asparagus

One cup of asparagus has 32.2 mg of calcium. In one spear of raw asparagus, the calcium content is 3 mg. Asparagus contain anti-inflammatory phytonutrients, antioxidant nutrients, including vitamin C, beta-carotene, vitamin E, and the minerals zinc, manganese, and selenium.

Ingredients:

- 3 lbs. Fresh mussels, rinsed, scrubbed and debearded (coarse thread on the side removed)
- 2 cups Asparagus, sliced into 1"
- 2 Tbsp. Garlic
- 3 Tbsp. Basil
- 2 Tbsp. Green onion
- 2 Tbsp. Fish sauce
- ¼ cup Olive oil
- Pepper to taste

Preparation:

Over high heat, sauté garlic in olive oil until brown. Add the mussels and asparagus. Stir-fry until mussel shells have started to open and asparagus is crisp yet tender. This will take around 5-7 minutes. Stir in the fish sauce. Discard mussels that have not opened. Add the basil and the green onion. Continue stirring for about a minute or until green onions are dark green. Add pepper to taste. Remove from heat and transfer to plate.

Amount Per Serving:

Serves: 5 • Serving size: 352 g

Calories 335

Total Fat 15.4g, Cholesterol 101 mg

Sodium 1402mg, potassium 1028mg

Total carbohydrates 13.7g, sugars 1.4g

Protein 34.3g

Vitamin A 25 % • Vitamin C 44% • Calcium 10 % •

Iron 67 %

14.   Creamy coconut meat fruit salad

Coconuts are highly nutritious and rich in, vitamins C, E, B1, B3, B5, B6, dietary fibre and minerals such as calcium, magnesium, phosphorous, iron, selenium, and sodium. This can be a good substitute to cow's milk because coconut milk is lactose-free. It also contains significant amount of fat and lauric acid that is converted to monalaurin which has antibacterial and antiviral properties.

Ingredients:

- 1 cup Coconut meat, shredded

- 1/2 cup Strawberries, halved

- ½ cup Grapes

- 1/2 cup Blueberries

- 1/2 cup Apple, diced

- 1/2 cup Pineapple, diced

- 1 kiwi, chopped

- 400 g. Canned sweetened condensed milk

- 400 g. Evaporated milk

Preparation:

Wash fruits thoroughly. Chop the Strawberries, apple, pineapple and kiwi. Throw all ingredients in a large bowl, stir, chill and enjoy!

Amount Per Serving:

Serves: 5 • Serving size: 257 g

Calories 463

Total Fat 18.6g, Cholesterol 50mg

Sodium 191mg, potassium 742mg

Total carbohydrates 64.7 g, sugars 60.3g

Protein12.9 g

Vitamin A 9% • Vitamin C 64% • Calcium 45% • Iron 17%

15.   Creamy butternut squash soup

Butternut squash is one of the most common varieties of winter squash. One cup of butternut squash provides 437% percent vitamin A requirement for the day, 52% of vitamin C, 10% or more of vitamin E, 7% of calcium and 5% of iron. It contains vitamin B-6, magnesium, niacin, thiamin, folate, pantothenic acid, and manganese. It is used to lower blood pressure, to prevent asthma, manage diabetes, prevent cancer and promotes healthy looking skin and hair.

Ingredients:

- 3 cups Butternut squash, cubed
- 1 Tbsp. Garlic
- ¼ cup Fresh ginger, sliced in large chunks
- 1 Tbsp. Onion, diced
- 2 Tbsp. Olive oil
- 2 cups Chicken stock
- ½ cup Heavy cream
- Salt and pepper to taste

Preparation:

Over medium heat, sauté garlic, ginger and onion in olive oil until translucent. Add the squash and stir for about a minute or two. Pour the chicken stock and bring to boil.

Lower the heat and simmer until squash is tender. Cool and puree in batches. Add the heavy cream and season with salt and pepper to taste. Enjoy!

Amount Per Serving:

Serves: 3 • Serving size: 346 g

Calories 249

Total Fat 17.7g, Cholesterol 27mg

Sodium 525mg, potassium 631mg

Total carbohydrates 23.8g, sugars 4.0 g

Protein 3.1 g

Vitamin A 304% • Vitamin C 52% • Calcium 10% • Iron 11%

16.   Cheesy turkey and avocado fried egg sandwich

One cup of pureed avocado has 27.6mg of calcium and 7 mg of dietary fiber. It contains high amount of good fatty acids, protein and vitamin K, which works in synergy with Vitamin D to help regulate osteoclast. It contains vitamin C, crucial for the production of collagen—a protein that promotes healthy bones and cartilage. It also contains boron involved in bone metabolism and vitamin D that regulates the amount of urinary calcium and magnesium excretion.

Ingredients:

- 2 slices Whole wheat bread

- 1 Tbsp. Avocado, peeled, pitted and mashed

- 1 Egg, fried

- 70 g. Leftover turkey, shredded

- ½ tsp. Mayonnaise

- 1 slice Gruyere cheese

Preparation:

In a small bowl, mix the turkey with mayonnaise. Set aside.

Spread avocado on both slices of wheat bread. Layer with fried egg, turkey with mayonnaise and cheese on a slice of bread. Cover the sandwich with another slice of whole wheat bread and enjoy!

Amount Per Serving:

Serves: 1 • Serving size: 116 g

Calories 294

Total Fat 23.4 g, Cholesterol 226mg

Sodium 562 mg, potassium 208mg

Total carbohydrates 2.3g, sugars g

Protein 18.8 g

Vitamin A 13% • Vitamin C 3% • Calcium 32 % • Iron 7 %

17.   Beef in tomato and celery soup

Two cups of raw celery have 81 mg of calcium. Celery contains a unique non-starch polysaccharide, which is responsible for its anti-inflammatory property. It is also rich in antioxidants like vitamin C and flavonoids.

Ingredients:

- 1 cup Celery, minced
- 200 g. Beef, minced
- 1 onion, chopped
- 2 cups Vegetable stock
- 2 400g. cans Diced tomatoes
- 1 Tbsp. Basil

Preparation:

Over medium heat, sauté the celery and onion in olive oil until onion is translucent. Add the minced beef and stir-fry until uniformly brown. Pour in the cans of diced tomatoes and vegetable stock. Stir and simmer for 5 minutes or until it lightly boils.

Amount Per Serving:

 Serves: 2• Serving size: 207g

Calories 216

Total Fat 6.4g, Cholesterol 89mg

Sodium 109 mg, potassium 618 mg

Total carbohydrates 6.7 g, sugars3.0 g

Protein 31.1g

Vitamin A 6% • Vitamin C 9% • Calcium 4% • Iron 106%

18.   Herb roasted chicken with leeks

One cup of leek has 52.5 mg calcium. It has a unique combination of flavonoids and sulfur-containing nutrient, called allium, which are known to possess antioxidant properties that protect against heart disease and cancer.

Ingredients:

- 6 pcs. Chicken drumsticks
- 2 Tbsp. Garlic
- 2 Tbsp. Onion
- 1 cup Leeks
- 1 cup Carrots
- 2 Tbsp. Flour
- 1 Tbsp. Thyme
- 1 Tbsp. Parsley
- ½ cup Olive oil
- ½ cup White wine

Preparation:

Preheat the oven to 450.

In a 9x13 inch baking dish, toss the garlic, onions, leeks, carrots, thyme and parsley and slather in olive oil. Season with salt and pepper.

Lightly rub the chicken legs with olive oil and season with thyme, salt and pepper. Arrange on top of the vegetables. Pour the white wine. Bake for about 35 to 40 minutes. When the chicken is done, any juices will run clear.

Amount Per Serving:

Serves: 2 • Serving size: 234 g

Calories 568

Total Fat 50.7 g, Cholesterol 0mg

Sodium 52mg, potassium 359mg

Total carbohydrates 21.2g, sugars 5.4 g

Protein 2.3 g

Vitamin A 203% • Vitamin C 21% • Calcium 8% • Iron 19%

19. Chocolate-almond oatmeal cookie with pumpkin seeds

One cup of pumpkin seed has 35.2 mg. of calcium and 262 mg. magnesium. Pumpkin seeds are a good source of vitamin B-complex, thiamin, niacin, folates, and pantothenic acid. The chemical component L-tryptophan also helps regulate mood.

Ingredients:

- 1 1/2 cup Pumpkin seeds, pureed
- 1/2 cup Almond paste
- 1 cup Olive oil
- 2 Tbsp. Extra Virgin Olive Oil
- 2 cups Honey
- 1 Egg yolk
- 1 tsp. Vanilla Extract
- 1 ¼ cups Flour
- ½ tsp. Salt
- 1 tsp. baking soda
- 3 cups Old fashioned rolled oats (not instant)
- 1 cup Cocoa powder

Preparation:

To puree the pumpkin seeds, roast the seeds in extra virgin olive oil over low-medium heat for 15-25 minutes or until seeds become light brown. Stir seeds every 10 minutes. Cool and transfer to a food processor. Blend for 5 minutes until consistency is smooth.

Preheat the oven to 350F.

Using an electric mixer, beat the olive oil, honey, almond paste and pumpkin seed puree. This should take around 7 minutes. Add the egg yolk and the vanilla extract. Continue beating until consistency of the mixture is smooth. In a separate bowl, mix together the oatmeal, flour, salt, baking soda and the cocoa powder. Slowly add 1/3 of the dry mixture to the wet mixture. Stir slowly using hand. Do not overmix. Continue adding the next 1/3, and finish by stirring in the remaining 1/3. Scoop out the cookies using a tablespoon and place them on a nonstick cookie sheet. Bake the cookies for 10-12 minutes or until edges are slightly brown.

Amount Per Serving:

Serves: 12 • Serving size: 97 g

Calories 461

Total Fat 29.7 g, Cholesterol 18mg

Sodium 209mg, potassium 394mg

Total carbohydrates 47.7 g, sugars 29.8 g

Protein 8.1g

Vitamin A 11% • Vitamin C 1% • Calcium 6% • Iron 26%

20.   Orange-honey glazed chicken

One cup of an orange juice contains 27.3 mg of calcium. While a one piece medium-sized fruit contains 65 mg. A study published in "Nutrition Research" in August 2005, found that the absorption of calcium from fat-free milk and calcium-fortified orange juice was basically the same at 35 percent and 36 percent, respectively.

Ingredients:

- 2 cups Chicken, cubed

- 2 Oranges, juiced

- ¼ cup Fish sauce

- 1/2 cup Honey

- 1 Tbsp. Garlic, minced

- 1 Tbsp, Ginger, minced

- 1 Tbsp. Onion leek

- 1/8 tsp. Pepper

- 1 cup Jasmine rice

Preparation:

In a skillet, over medium heat, combine the chicken, honey, orange juice, fish sauce, garlic, ginger and pepper. Cook and stir until the chicken is well-cooked and the sauce is sticky glazed, or for about 20 minutes. Throw in the onion leeks, stir and cook for another minute before removing from fire. Enjoy with a cup of rice.

Amount Per Serving:

Serves: 4 • Serving size: 201 g

Calories 343

Total Fat 0.1 g, Cholesterol 0mg

Sodium 1392mg, potassium 252mg

Total carbohydrates 83.3g, sugars 44.1 g

Protein 5.1g

Vitamin A 5% • Vitamin C 83% • Calcium 5% • Iron 11%

21.   Red velvet with sunflower seeds muffin

One cup of sunflower seeds contains 400 mg of calcium. It also contains protein, dietary fibers and mono and poly-unsaturated fats. It is also rich in potassium, magnesium and selenium.

Ingredients:

- 1/2 cup sunflower seeds
- 1/4 cup Olive oil
- 1 cup Honey
- 1 egg
- 1 ¼ Tbsp. Cocoa powder
- 1 tsp. Red food coloring
- 1 1/4 cups Flour
- 1/2 tsp. Salt
- 1 tsp. Vanilla extract
- 1/2 cup milk
- ½ Tbsp. Vinegar
- 2 Tbsp. Water
- 1/2 tsp. Lemon juice
- 1/2 tsp. Baking soda

Cream cheese icing:

- 4 oz. Cream cheese
- 1/4 cup Olive oil
- ¾ Tbsp. Stevia
- 1/2 tsp. Vanilla extract

Preparation:

Preheat the oven to 350F.

Place liners on the muffin tin.

Using an electric mixer, blend the honey and olive oil. Add the egg and blend well. In a small bowl, combine the cocoa powder and the red food coloring. Mix before transferring to the mixing bowl containing the olive oil and honey mixture. Sift the flour and salt. Transfer to the mixing bowl and mix. Add the vanilla, milk, vinegar, and water into the mixing bowl. In a separate bowl, combine and mix the lemon juice and baking soda before transferring to the mixing bowl with the batter. Pour the batter evenly into the liners. Bake for 25 minutes.

To make the cream cheese icing, combine all ingredients and blend well using an electric mixer. Spread on top of the cooled cupcakes.

Amount Per Serving:

Serves: 6 • Serving size: 153 g

Calories 526

Total Fat 25.2g, Cholesterol 90 mg

Sodium 496mg, potassium 151mg

Total carbohydrates 71.2g, sugars 49.4 g

Protein 6.9g

Vitamin A 15% • Vitamin C 1 % • Calcium 6% • Iron 11%

22.   Cinnamon apple crumble

Cinnamon slows down bone breakdown and prevents osteoporotic bone loss. One tablespoon of cinnamon contains 78.2 mg of calcium. Cinnamon is also rich in fiber and in manganese.

Ingredients:

- 6 Apples, diced
- 2/3 cup Flour
- 2/3 cup Honey
- 1 tsp. Salt
- 1 Tbsp. Cinnamon
- 6 Tbsp. Olive oil
- 1 Tbsp. Olive oil

Preparation:

Preheat the oven in 350F and grease an 8x9 inches baking dish with olive oil.

Place the apples in a baking dish.

To make the crumble topping, in a medium bowl, whisk in the flour, honey, salt and cinnamon. Add the olive oil. Knead using hands until mixture is crumbly and sandy. Do not overmix.

Amount Per Serving:

Serves: 8 • Serving size: 173 g

Calories 248

Total Fat 10.7 g, Cholesterol 23mg

Sodium 356mg, potassium 176mg

Total carbohydrates 39.4g, sugars 26.0g

Protein1.6 g

Vitamin A 5% • Vitamin C 17% • Calcium 2% • Iron 7%

Place the crumble topping on top of the apples, completely covering it. Bake for 45 minutes until 1 hour or until top is golden brown and apples are cooked completely.

23.   Chicken salad with mushrooms in sesame seed dressing

Sesame seeds are an excellent source of magnesium, copper, calcium, phosphorous, iron, zinc, molybdenum and selenium. A tablespoon of sesame seeds with the hulk removed contains 37 mg of calcium. Zinc helps increase the bone mineral density.

Ingredients:

- 1 Tbsp. Toasted sesame seeds, grounded
- ½ cup Chicken breast fillet, cubed
- 1 medium head Romaine lettuce
- 1 cup Spinach
- ¾ cup Shiitake mushroom, sliced thinly
- 1/2 cup Tomatoes, chopped
- 1 Tbsp. Onions, chopped
- 1 Tbsp. Olive oil
- Salt and pepper to taste

Salad dressing

- ½ Tbsp. Sesame oil
- ½ Tbsp. Olive oil
- ½ cup Dashi

- 1/3 cup Fish sauce

- 2 Tbsp. Honey

Preparation:

In a small bowl make the salad dressing by mixing sesame oil, olive oil, dashi, fish sauce and honey.

In a medium sized bowl, mix all vegetables.

Season the chicken and shiitake mushroom with salt and pepper and sauté together with onions in olive oil over medium heat. Cook until onion is translucent and chicken is thoroughly cooked. Remove from fire and toss into the salad.

Drizzle the sesame seed dressing on top of the salad and enjoy!

Amount Per Serving:

 Serves: 2 • Serving size: 395 g

Calories 371

Total Fat 21.5g, Cholesterol 31mg

Sodium 2580mg, potassium 710mg

Total carbohydrates 32.5 g, sugars 17.8 g

Protein 16.9 g

Vitamin A 36 % • Vitamin C 30% • Calcium 13% • Iron 43%

24.   Roast beef with watercress sandwich

Watercress is believed to cleanse the blood. It has more iron than spinach, more vitamin C than oranges, and more calcium than a glass of milk. It can also inhibit carcinogens and contains phytonutrients which help prevent disease.

Ingredients:

- 3 oz. Sirloin tip, thinly sliced
- 1 tsp. Olive oil
- 1 Large white onion, sliced into rings
- 1/8 tsp. Garlic powder
- Salt and pepper
- ¼ cup Watercress
- 1 large white onion, sliced into rings.
- 1 French bread
- 4 oz. Provolone cheese, thinly sliced

Preparation:

Lightly rub the roast beef with olive oil and season with garlic powder, salt and pepper. Toast inside an oven in 250 F for 10 minutes.

Over medium heat, sauté the onion in olive oil until slightly brown. Season with salt and pepper.

Cut open the French bread into half. Place the roast beef on top of the bread, layer with watercress followed by caramelized onion, then cheese. Broil for 2 minutes until cheese is melted. Serve and enjoy!

Amount Per Serving:

Serves: 2 • Serving size: 214g

Calories 281

Total Fat 17.6g, Cholesterol 39mg

Sodium 505mg, potassium 308mg

Total carbohydrates 15.4g, sugars 6.7g

Protein 16.3g

Vitamin A 11% • Vitamin C 21% • Calcium 46% • Iron 4%

25.   Chicken curry with green papaya

Papaya is rich in vitamin C which functions to remove free radicals from the body, boosts the immune system and functions as an anti-inflammatory. It is also rich in vitamin K which helps in calcium absorption and reduces the excretion of calcium in the urine.

Ingredients:

- 500 g. Chicken breast fillet, cut into strips

- 2 cups Green papaya, sliced into 2"

- 2 Tsp. Curry powder

- 2 Tbsp. Vegetable oil

- 1 Onion, finely chopped

- 2 Tbsp. Garlic, minced

- 1 Tbsp. Ginger

- 2 cups Chicken broth

- 2 cups Coconut milk

- 1 cup Jasmine rice, cooked

Preparation:

Over medium heat, sauté the garlic until brown and onion until translucent. Add the curry powder and throw in the chicken. Cook until light brown or for about 5-7 minutes.

Add the papaya, chicken broth and the coconut milk. Lower the heat and simmer until sauce is creamy and thick or for about 10 minutes. Season with salt and pepper to taste. Best enjoyed with rice.

Amount Per Serving:

Serves: 6 • Serving size: 301 g

Calories 519

Total Fat 30.4g, Cholesterol 74mg

Sodium 340mg, potassium 542mg

Total carbohydrates 32.4 g, sugars 3.8g

Protein 30.1g

Vitamin A 1% • Vitamin C 8% • Calcium 4% • Iron 21%

26.   Cream dory with Swiss chard

Swiss chard provides excellent bone support because of calcium, magnesium and vitamin K. Vitamin K1 in particular, prevents excessive activation of osteoclasts cells, which is responsible for bone break down. Additionally, friendly bacteria present in the intestines convert vitamin K1 into vitamin K2, which activates osteocalcin, the major non-collagen protein in the bone.

Ingredients:

- 1 Tbsp. Olive oil
- 2 Tbsp. Garlic
- 4 Cream dory fillets
- 12 cups Swiss chard leaves, cut into 2" pieces
- 2 Tbsp. Lemon juice
- 2 Tbsp. Olive oil
- 1/8 tsp. Salt
- 1/8 tsp. Pepper

Preparation:

Lightly season the cream dory fillet with olive oil, salt and pepper.

In a pan, over medium-heat, sauté garlic in olive oil until brown. Add the cream dory fillets and cook until light brown on both sides or for about 2 minutes on each side. Add the lemon juice. Throw in the Swiss chard leaves and cook until wilted or for about 4 minutes. Season with salt and pepper.

Amount Per Serving:

Serves: 2 • Serving size: 262g

Calories 229

Total Fat 20.5 g, Cholesterol 15mg

Sodium 655mg, potassium 876mg

Total carbohydrates 11.3g, sugars 2.8g

Protein 4.6g

Vitamin A 268% • Vitamin C 124% • Calcium 13% • Iron 23%

27.   Sweet Asian kelp noodles

Kelp absorbs numerous nutrients from its surrounding marine environment. This is why it is very rich in vitamins, trace elements, enzymes and minerals. Kelp is known to have more calcium than kale or collard greens.

Ingredients:

- 1 package Kelp noodles, softened by washing
- 1/4 cup gluten-free tamari
- 1/2 cup vegetable broth
- 1 Tbsp. rice wine vinegar
- 1 Tbsp. Sesame oil
- 1 Tbsp. Sesame seeds
- 1 tsp. Cornstarch
- 3 Tbsp.Honey
- 1 small onion, diced
- ¼ cup Onion leeks, chopped
- 1 Tbsp. Garlic, minced
- ¼ cup Ginger, peeled then grated
- ½ cup Green bell pepper, sliced thinly
- 1 cup Watercress
- 1 /2 cup Carrot

- 1 cup Shiitake mushrooms, sliced

Preparation:

Heat a wok over high heat. Stir fry the garlic, onions, leeks and bell peppers for 3 minutes. Add the ginger, carrots, watercress and mushroom. Stir until vegetables are tender. Add in the tamari, vegetable broth, cornstarch, honey, rice wine vinegar and sesame oil. Stir well. Reduce the heat and stir continuously until sauce is thickened, or for about 2 minutes. Toss in the kelp noodles and sprinkle with sesame seeds. Enjoy while hot!

Amount Per Serving:

Serves: 3 • Serving size: 324 g

Calories 256

Total Fat 7.5g, Cholesterol 0mg

Sodium1843 mg, potassium 512mg

Total carbohydrates 43.3 g, sugars 18.0g

Protein 8.1g

Vitamin A 80% • Vitamin C 56% • Calcium 24% • Iron 30%

28.   Banana cake

Banana is rich in a carbohydrate called fructooligosaccharides, which allows increase in the production of digestive enzymes and vitamins that help absorb important bone-strengthening nutrients such as calcium and magnesium.

Ingredients:

- 3 cups Flour
- 2 2/3 cups Blackstrap molasses
- 1 cup Olive oil
- 4 Ripe bananas, mashed
- 1/4 cup milk
- 2 Eggs
- 1 tsp. vanilla extract

Preparation:

Preheat the oven to 350F.

Mix the honey and olive oil until well blended. Mash or puree the banana using a food processor. Transfer to the olive oil and honey mixture. In a small bowl, whisk the eggs. Pour into the mixing bowl. Mix all the remaining ingredients. Blend well until consistency is thick but smooth. Pour the mixture into the greased 9 inches round pan. Bake for 40 minutes.

Amount Per Serving:

Serves: 12 • Serving size: 175 g

Calories 510

Total Fat 16.7g, Cholesterol 28mg

Sodium 41mg, potassium 1255mg

Total carbohydrates 87.7 g, sugars 45.7g

Protein 4.8g

Vitamin A 11% • Vitamin C 6% • Calcium17 % • Iron 28%

29.   Turkey with kale laden with walnut sauce

One cup of cooked kale has 1,062 mg. of vitamin K, more than 1,300% of the recommended daily value. Vitamin K is important in healthy bone remodeling. Vitamin K, in conjunction with vitamin D, regulates osteoclast production.

Ingredients:

- 1 lb. Kale
- 300g. Turkey
- 1 Tbsp. Garlic, finely chopped
- 2 Tbsp. Onion, chopped
- 1 Tbsp. Olive oil
- Salt to taste

Walnut Sauce:

- 1 slice French bread, crusts removed
- ½ cup Milk
- 3 cups walnuts
- 2 Tbsp. Garlic, minced
- 2 Tbsp. Onion, finely diced
- 1 Tbsp. paprika

- 1/4 tsp. Cayenne pepper

- 2 cups Turkey stock

- Salt

Preparation:

Boil turkey for 2-3 hours over low heat. Strain the stock and set aside. Shred the turkey and set aside.

Steam the kale until tender or for about 10 minutes. Drain well.

To make the walnut sauce, soak the bread in milk. Blend the soaked bread with walnuts, garlic, onion, salt, cayenne, paprika and strained turkey stock. Mix well and blend by batches until consistency is smooth.

In a large skillet over medium heat sauté garlic in olive oil until brown. Add kale to the skillet. Cook until leaves are wilted or for about 5 minutes. Throw in the shredded turkey. Stir for a while. Transfer to a plate and pour walnut sauce on top. Enjoy!

Amount Per Serving:

Serves: 10 • Serving size: 137 g

Calories 340

Total Fat 25.5g, Cholesterol 24mg

Sodium 115mg, potassium 553mg

Total carbohydrates12.5 g, sugars 1.3g

Protein 20.2 g

Vitamin A 148 % • Vitamin C 94% • Calcium 11% •

Iron29 %

30.   Blackberry maple syrup crepe

Like spinach, plums and apples, blackberries are rich in bioflavonoids and vitamin C. Its dark colour suggests that it contains a high amount of antioxidant. It also contains high amount of calcium, and magnesium that helps in calcium and potassium absorption in the body. The phosphorous aids in regulating calcium and aids in building strong bones and proper cellular functioning.

Ingredients:

- 1/2 cup. Blackberry
- 1 cup Flour
- 2 Eggs
- 1 cup Milk
- 1/4 cup Water
- 4 Tbsp. Olive oil
- 4 Tbsp. Maple syrup
- ½ cup Honey
- 1/8 tsp. Salt

Preparation:

Combine blackberries and maple syrup in a small saucepan over medium heat. Remove from heat. Cool.

Whisk the eggs and salt. Slowly add the milk and alternate with flour. Mix well. Whisk in the honey and olive oil.

Grease an 8 "diameter non-stick skillet and place on top of stove over medium heat. Scoop about ¼ cup of batter and place in the middle of the pan. Spread it thinly and evenly by lifting the pan and gently moving your hand in a circular motion to swirl the batter. Using a spatula, gently flip the crepe to the other side once a fine lace pattern is seen. Do not overcook crepe. Place the blackberries in maple syrup in the center of the crepe. Fold in half and transfer to a warm plate.

Amount Per Serving:

 Serves: 4 • Serving size: 163 g

Calories 330

Total Fat 15.3g, Cholesterol 117mg

Sodium 218mg, potassium 142mg

Total carbohydrates 40.5g, sugars 14.9g

Protein 8.1g

Vitamin A 10% • Vitamin C 0% • Calcium 11% • Iron 12%

31.   Green turnips soup

Turnip greens is filled with folate, antioxidants and calcium. The noticeably bitter taste of turnip greens is associated with its presence of concentrated amount of calcium in varying forms such as calcium chloride, calcium sulfate, calcium lactate, calcium pectate and other forms.

Ingredients:

- 1 tsp. Vegetable oil
- 1 lb. Smoked sausage, thinly sliced
- 4 Tbsp. Onion, chopped
- 5 cups Chicken broth
- 2 20oz. canned Turnip greens
- 2 14 oz. canned Cannellini beans
- 1 package Vegetable soup mix
- 1 tsp. Hot pepper sauce
- 1 tsp. Garlic powder
- Salt and pepper to taste

Preparation:

In a skillet over medium heat, brown the sausage lightly in vegetable oil. Add all other ingredients and simmer until desired flavor is reached or for about 30 minutes. Serve hot and enjoy!

Amount Per Serving:

Serves: 12 • Serving size: 311 g

Calories 400

Total Fat 12.5g, Cholesterol 32mg

Sodium 655mg, potassium 1414mg

Total carbohydrates47.3 g, sugars 2.7g

Protein 26.5g

Vitamin A 219% • Vitamin C 100% • Calcium 28% • Iron 40%

32.   Banana date nut bread

Brown dates have a good nutritional value, and are usually packed with all-natural fibers, vitamins and minerals. It is very low in calories and zero in cholesterol.

Ingredients:

- 3 Ripe bananas, mashed
- 1/2 cup Brown dates, chopped into small pieces
- 1/2 cup Walnut
- 2 cups Honey
- 3/4 cup Olive oil
- 1½ cups Flour
- 3 Eggs
- 6 Tbsp. Milk
- 1 tsp. Vanilla extract

Preparation:

Preheat the oven to 350F.

 Beat the olive oil and honey until smooth. Add the eggs and milk. Add the flour and beat well. Add the vanilla, bananas, brown dates and walnuts. Mix until consistency is smooth. Transfer to a greased pan and bake for 1 hour.

Amount Per Serving:

Serves: 8 • Serving size: 186   g

Calories 575

Total Fat 14.2g, Cholesterol 108mg

Sodium 152mg, potassium 332mg

Total carbohydrates 87.9g, sugars63.3 g

Protein7.7 g

Vitamin A 13% • Vitamin C 7% • Calcium 4% • Iron 10%

33.   Quick peanut butter cinnamon raisin sandwich

Raisin is a very good source of boron, a micronutrient that is vital in proper bone formation and efficient calcium absorption. Boron is particularly helpful in preventing osteoporosis among menopausal women and has been shown to help prevent bone and joint disease.

Ingredients:

- 2 slices Whole wheat bread
- 1 1/2 Tbsp. Peanut butter
- 1 tsp Raisin
- 1/8 tsp. Cinnamon

Preparation:

In a small mixing bowl, combine all ingredients and mix well. Spread generously on a slice of wheat bread and enjoy!

Amount Per Serving:

Serves: 1 • Serving size: 83 g

Calories 289

Total Fat14.0g, Cholesterol 0mg

Sodium 375mg, potassium 319mg

Total carbohydrates 30.5g, sugars 7.2g

Protein 13.3g

Vitamin A 0% • Vitamin C 0% • Calcium7 % • Iron 21%

34.   Stir-fried chicken noodles with figs

Dried figs have a high concentration of calcium, potassium, fiber and sugar. Just two of these treat provide 55 mg. of bone-healthy calcium, accounting for almost 6% of the daily average need.

Ingredients:

- 350 g. Egg noodles
- 300g. Chicken, cut in strips
- 3/4 cup Onions, chopped
- 1 Tbsp. Green onions
- 4 Tbsp. Olive oil
- 10 Dried figs, coarsely chopped
- 3/4 cup Honey
- 3 Tbsp. Lemon juice
- 2 Tbsp. Garlic, minced
- 1 tsp. Salt
- 1 tsp. Paprika

Preparation:

Cook noodles according to package instructions. Drain noodles and set aside.

In a large skillet, over medium heat, sauté onions in olive oil until translucent. Add the chicken and cook until light brown. Add the garlic, figs, honey, lemon juice, and salt. Bring to a boil. Lower fire, cover pan with a lid and simmer for 20 minutes or until mixture is thick. Add the green onions and paprika then stir. Toss in the noodles, stir and serve.

Amount Per Serving:

Serves: 10 • Serving size: 131 g

Calories 264

Total Fat 6.7g, Cholesterol 44mg

Sodium 289mg, potassium 315mg

Total carbohydrates 43.5g, sugars 30.6g

Protein 10.5g

Vitamin A 5% • Vitamin C 6% • Calcium 5% • Iron 7%

35.   Banana walnut raisin oatmeal

Oatmeal makes an ideal breakfast meal because it is filling and it provides numerous health benefits. It is packed with fiber and calcium. A cup of oatmeal contains 187.2 mg of calcium.

Ingredients:

- 1 1/2 cup Rolled oatmeal
- 1/8 tsp. Cinnamon
- 1 tsp. Raisin
- 2 tsp. Crumbled walnuts
- 1/2 cup Banana, sliced
- 1 cup Water
- 1 cup Milk
- 2 Tbsp. maple syrup

Preparation:

Boil oats in water and milk. Simmer and stir often. Transfer to a bowl and toss in all ingredients.

Amount Per Serving:

Serves: 4 • Serving size: 182 g

Calories 200

Total Fat 4.1g, Cholesterol 5mg

Sodium 34mg, potassium247 mg

Total carbohydrates 35.5g, sugars 11.8g

Protein 6.6g

Vitamin A 1% • Vitamin C 3% • Calcium 10% • Iron 9%

36.   Prickly pear with Apple and strawberry smoothie

Prickly pears contain a high amount of calcium. It is high in vitamin C, B complex, magnesium, copper, dietary fiber and potassium. Prickly pears have high levels of flavonoids, polyphenols and betalains.

Ingredients:

- 1 cup Prickly peeled
- 3 cups Apples
- 1 cup Strawberries
- 1 cup Plain yogurt
- 1 cup Ice

Preparation:

Throw in all ingredients in a blender. Blend well and transfer into chilled glasses and enjoy!

Amount Per Serving:

Serves: 4 • Serving size: 179 g

Calories 98

Total Fat 1.0g, Cholesterol 4mg

Sodium 44mg, potassium 286mg

Total carbohydrates18.4 g, sugars 14.6g

Protein4.0 g

Vitamin A 1% • Vitamin C 46% • Calcium 12% • Iron3 %

37.   Chicken apricots salad

Apricot is rich in iron, vitamin A, C, beta-carotene, and potassium. The vitamin K present in apricots improves bone health while lowering the occurrence of bone fractures. Two ounces of dried apricots contain 52 mg. of calcium.

Ingredients:

- 200g. Leftover chicken, shredded
- 1 cup Apricot, cubed
- 1/2 cup Pecan
- 1 medium head Romaine lettuce
- 3/4 cup Potatoes, steamed and cubed
- Dressing
- 3/4 cup Mayonnaise
- 1/4 cup Mustard
- 2 Tbsp. Honey

Preparation:

To make the dressing, mix all ingredients.

In a medium bowl, stir in all vegetables, apricot and pecan. Top with a salad dressing and enjoy!

Amount Per Serving:

Serves: 6 • Serving size: 175 g

Calories 250

Total Fat13.0 g, Cholesterol 33mg

Sodium 235mg, potassium 333mg

Total carbohydrates 22.5g, sugars11.2 g

Protein 12.5g

Vitamin A 12% • Vitamin C 15% • Calcium 5% • Iron 15%

38.   Creamy onion soup

In a research conducted at the University of Basel, they have observed that the onion peptide GPCS (γ-glutamyl-propenyl-cysteine sulfoxide) reduces bone breakdown in rats. The high amount of sulfur in onions affects the formation of connective tissues such as cartilage and tendon as well.

Ingredients:

- 4 cups Onions
- 2 Tbsp. Olive oil
- 2 Tbsp. Garlic
- 3 cups Chicken broth
- 1 Chicken bouillon cube
- 1 cup Cream
- 3 Tbsp. Flour
- 1 1/2 cup Milk
- 1/4 cup Cheddar cheese, shredded
- 1/8 tsp. Pepper

Preparation:

To make the white sauce, in a small saucepan, over medium heat, add olive oil then add flour until thick. Slowly pour milk in flour and stir constantly until mixture is thick. Stir in the cream. Set aside.

In a medium saucepan, over low to medium heat, cook garlic and onions in olive oil until tender. Stir frequently. Add chicken broth, bouillon cube, and pepper and stir occasionally.

 Add white sauce and Cheddar cheese to onion mixture. Simmer on medium low heat until the cheese is melted and all ingredients are blended, stirring occasionally. Lower heat and cook for another 30 to 45 minutes.

Amount Per Serving:

 Serves: 6 • Serving size: 281 g

Calories 151

Total Fat 6.5g, Cholesterol 19mg

Sodium 563mg, potassium 288mg

Total carbohydrates16.0 g, sugars 7.3g

Protein7.4 g

Vitamin A 3% • Vitamin C 10 % • Calcium 15% • Iron 4%

39.   Leche flan

Regular consumption of dairy is associated with lower rates of osteoporosis and better bone health. Milk contains high amount of phosphate which increases calcium retention and improves bone health.

Ingredients:

- 1 cup Maple syrup

- 7 eggs

- 400g Condensed milk

- 380g. Evaporated milk

Preparation:

Grease individual ramekins.

Stir together the condensed milk and the evaporated milk in a mixing bowl until they're thoroughly combined. Beat the eggs into the mixture, one at a time. The finished mixture should be light, fluffy and creamy. Add 1 tsp. Vanilla extract. Pour into the ramekins. Refrigerate and serve cool.

Amount Per Serving:

Serves: 8 • Serving size: 144 g

Calories 310

Total Fat 11.8g, Cholesterol 174mg

Sodium 168mg, potassium 381mg

Total carbohydrates 40.6g, sugars 40.6g

Protein 12.0g

Vitamin A 9% • Vitamin C 4% • Calcium 29% • Iron 5%

40.   Blueberry and yogurt pancake

One cup serving of yogurt contains 42% of the recommended daily amount of calcium. Yogurt is an excellent source of calcium, vitamins B2, B12, potassium and magnesium. It is rich in probiotics which improve the immune system.

Ingredients:

- 1 ½ cups Flour, all-purpose
- 2 Tbsp. Honey
- 120 mL Yogurt plain low-fat
- 1 cup Blueberries, frozen
- 2 tsp. Baking powder
- ½ tsp. Baking soda
- ½ tsp. salt
- 1 ½ cups Milk
- 2 Tbsp. Olive oil
- 2 Eggs

Preparation:

In a large bowl, combine and whisk the flour, baking powder, baking soda and salt. In a separate bowl, combine and mix the milk, eggs, yogurt, olive oil and cooking oil.

Combine with the flour and baking powder mixture. Mix well until batter is smooth. Add the frozen berries. On a griddle, over medium-high heat, heat the oil. Mix the batter first before scooping some batter onto the griddle. Fry the batter until light brown, or over two minutes, then flip onto the other side. Take the pancake off the griddle and transfer to a plate.

Amount Per Serving:

Serves: 4 • Serving size: 214 g

Calories 344

Total Fat 10.4 g, Cholesterol 105mg

Sodium 568mg, potassium 414mg

Total carbohydrates 52.9g, sugars14.0 g

Protein 11.0g

Vitamin A 6% • Vitamin C 10% • Calcium 24% • Iron 18%

41.   Vanilla with chia seeds

Chia seeds contain almost the same amount of calcium in a cup of milk. It is rich in omega-3 fatty acids that help lower the risk of heart disease and stroke. It also contains high amount of dietary fiber.

Ingredients:

- ½ cup Almond milk
- 2 Tbsp. Honey
- 1 Tbsp. Cocoa powder
- 1 Tbsp. Chia seeds
- 1 cup Ice
- 1 Tbsp. Vanilla extract
- Whipped cream for garnish

Preparation:

Boil almond milk with vanilla extract in 4 oz. water. Cool. Transfer to a blender along with the remaining ingredients. Transfer to a chilled glass and enjoy!

Amount Per Serving:

Serves: 2 • Serving size: 84 g

Calories 209

Total Fat 14.8g, Cholesterol 0mg

Sodium 10mg, potassium 237mg

Total carbohydrates 17.6g, sugars14.9 g

Protein 1.9g

Vitamin A 0% • Vitamin C 3% • Calcium 1% • Iron8 %

42.   Smoked salmon salad with dill

Ingredients:

- 1 cup Smoked salmon, thinly sliced
- 1 tsp Lemon juice
- 2 Tbsp. Olive oil
- 1 Tbsp. Dill
- 2 heads of Romaine lettuce

Preparation:

In a medium bowl, mix the dill, lemon juice and olive oil. Add the smoked salmon and mix until the salmon is completely covered in the olive oil mixture. Toss in the romaine lettuce, mix and enjoy!

Amount Per Serving:

Serves: 2 • Serving size: 343 g

Calories 169

Total Fat 14.7g, Cholesterol0 mg

Sodium 21mg, potassium 511mg

Total carbohydrates 10.6g, sugars 3.3g

Protein 1.8g

Vitamin A 2% • Vitamin C 28% • Calcium 3% • Iron 53%

JUICES

1.   Beet Banana Juice

Ingredients:

2 cups of beets

1 small banana, peeled

1 cup of blueberries, fresh

3 cups of beet greens, chopped

Preparation:

Wash the beets and separate the beet greens. Chop into small pieces and set aside.

Peel the banana and cut into chunks. Set aside.

Wash the blueberries under cold running water. Drain and set aside.

Now, process beets, beet greens, banana and blueberries in a juicer.

Transfer to serving glasses and serve immediately.

Nutritional information per serving: Kcal: 242, Protein: 9.1g, Carbs: 75.4g, Fats: 1.4g

2.   Blackberry Orange Juice

Ingredients:

1 cup of blackberries, fresh

1 large orange, peeled

2 wedges of watermelon, seeded

½ cup of pure coconut water, unsweetened

1 tbsp of honey, raw

Preparation:

Wash the blackberries under cold running water and set aside.

Peel the orange and divide into wedges. Set aside.

Cut the watermelon lengthwise. Cut two large wedges and peel them. Cut into chunks and remove the seeds. Set aside.

Now, combine blackberries, orange, and watermelon in a juicer and process until juiced.

Transfer to serving glasses and stir the coconut water and honey.

Refrigerate for 5 minutes before serving.

Enjoy!

Nutrition information per serving: Kcal: 264, Protein: 7.2g, Carbs: 78.6g, Fats: 1.7g

3.   Mint Celery Juice

Ingredients:

1 cup of avocado, sliced

1 tbsp of fresh mint, finely chopped

1 cup of celery, chopped

1 cup of green cabbage, torn

½ cup of pure coconut water, unsweetened

Preparation:

Peel the avocado and cut in half. Remove the pit and cut into chunks. Set aside.

Wash the celery and cut into small pieces. Set aside.

Wash the mint and cabbage thoroughly and torn with hands. Set aside.

Now, process mint, celery, avocado, and cabbage in a juicer and process until juiced.

Transfer to serving glasses and stir in coconut water. Garnish with fresh mint and add some ice.

Enjoy!

Nutritional information per serving: Kcal: 219, Protein: 4.8g, Carbs: 20.8g, Fats: 21.6g

4.   Lemon Cucumber Juice

Ingredients:

1 large lemon, peeled

4 cups of cucumber

3 large Granny Smith apples, cored

¼ cup of water

1 tbsp of liquid honey

Preparation:

Peel the lemon and cut lengthwise in half. Set aside.

Wash the cucumber and cut into thick slices. Set aside.

Wash the apples and remove the core. Cut into bite-sized pieces and set aside.

Now, combine lemon, cucumber, and apples in a juicer and process until juiced. Transfer to serving glasses and stir in the water and liquid honey.

Garnish with some fresh mint, but this is optional.

Add few ice cubes before serving and enjoy!

Nutrition information per serving: Kcal: 327, Protein: 4.7g, Carbs: 97g, Fats: 1.5g

5.   Grapefruit Lime Juice

Ingredients:

1 whole grapefruit, peeled

1 whole lime, peeled

2 cups of cherries, without pits

1 tbsp of fresh mint, chopped

Preparation:

Peel the grapefruit and divide into wedges. Set aside.

Peel the lime and cut lengthwise in half. Set aside.

Wash the cherries under cold running water. Cut in half and remove the pits. Set aside.

Now, process cherries, grapefruit, and lime in a juicer and process until juiced.Transfer to serving glasses and garnish with fresh mint.

Enjoy!

Nutritional information per serving: Kcal: 266, Protein: 5.3g, Carbs: 79.4g, Fats: 1g

6.   Pear Cabbage Juice

Ingredients:

1 large pear, cored

1 cup of green cabbage, roughly chopped

4 cups of crookneck squash, sliced

½ cup of pure coconut water, unsweetened

Preparation:

Wash the pear and remove the core. Cut into bite-sized pieces and set aside.

Wash the cabbage thoroughly and roughly chop it. Set aside.

Wash the crookneck squash and cut in half. Scoop out the seeds using a spoon. Cut into small chunks and set aside. Reserve the rest for another juice.

Now, combine pear, green cabbage, and crookneck squash in a juicer and process until juiced.

Transfer to serving glasses and stir in the coconut water.

Add some ice and serve immediately.

Nutritional information per serving: Kcal: 192, Protein: 7g, Carbs: 59.9g, Fats: 1.7g

7.   Coconut Berry Juice

Ingredients:

1 cup of blueberries

1 cup of strawberries

1 cup of cranberries

1 cup of raspberries

1 cup of blackberries

1 small granny Smith apple

¼ cup of water

1 tsp of pure coconut sugar

2 oz of water

Preparation:

Combine all berries in a colander and wash under cold running water. Cut the strawberries in half and set aside.

Soak the berries in water for 5 minutes. Drain and set aside.

Wash the apple and remove the core. Cut into bite-sized pieces and set aside. Now, process all berries and apple in a juicer.Transfer to serving glasses and stir in the coconut sugar and water. Add some ice and serve!

Nutrition information per serving: Kcal: 210, Protein: 5.7g, Carbs: 82g, Fats: 2.4g

8.   Kiwi Kale Juice

Ingredients:

4 kiwis, peeled

2 cups of kale, torn

1 cup of mango, chopped

1 tbsp of fresh mint, finely chopped

Preparation:

Peel the kiwis and cut lengthwise in half. Set aside.

Wash the kale thoroughly and torn with hands. Set aside.

Wash the mango and cut into small chunks. Set aside.

Now, combine kiwis, kale, and mango in a juicer and process until juiced.

Transfer to serving glasses and add few ice cubes. Garnish with fresh mint and serve immediately.

Nutritional information per serving: Kcal: 272, Protein: 10.3g, Carbs: 77g, Fats: 3.3g

9.   Cucumber Ginger Juice

Ingredients:

1 large cucumber

1 ginger root knob, 1-inch

1 cup of sweet potatoes, cubed

1 cup of spinach, torn

Preparation:

Wash the cucumber and cut into thick slices. Set aside.

Peel the ginger root knob and set aside.

Peel the sweet potatoes and cut into small cubes. Fill the measuring cup and reserve the rest for some other juice. Set aside.

Wash the spinach thoroughly under cold running water and torn with hands. Set aside.

Now, combine cucumber,ginger, sweet potatoes, and spinach in a juicer and process until juiced.

Transfer to serving glasses stir in the water. Refrigerate for 5 minutes before serving.

Nutrition information per serving: Kcal: 190, Protein: 13.8g, Carbs: 51.1g, Fats: 1.7g

10.   Strawberry Apple Juice

Ingredients:

1 cup of strawberries

1 large green apple, cored

3 large peaches, pitted

¼ tsp of ginger, ground

Preparation:

Wash the strawberries and cut into halves. Set aside.

Wash the apple and remove the core. Cut into bite-sized pieces and set aside.

Wash the peaches and cut into halves. Remove the pits and set aside.

Now, combine strawberries, apple, and peaches in a juicer. Process until juiced. Transfer to serving glasses and stir in the ginger.

Refrigerate for 10 minutes before serving.

Enjoy!

Nutritional information per serving: Kcal: 64, Protein: 1.2g, Carbs: 18.3g, Fats: 0.1g

11.   Watercress Lime Juice

Ingredients:

1 cup of watercress, chopped

1 whole lime, peeled

1 cup of watermelon, diced

1 slice of ginger

1 cup of blueberries

Preparation:

Wash the watercress thoroughly and roughly chop it. Set aside.

Peel the lime and cut lengthwise in half. Set aside.

Cut the watermelon lengthwise. For one cup, you will need about 1 large wedge. Peel and cut into chunks. Remove the seeds and set aside. Reserve the rest of for some other juices.

Peel the ginger slice and set aside.

Wash the blueberries under cold running water and set aside.

Now, process watercress, lime, watermelon, ginger, and blueberries in a juicer.

Transfer to serving glasses and add some ice.

Serve immediately.

Nutritional information per serving: Kcal: 129, Protein: 3g, Carbs: 37.4g, Fats: 0.8g

12.   Blackberry Grape Juice

Ingredients:

1 cup of fresh blackberries

1 cup of black grapes

1 cup of fresh strawberries

1 medium-sized green apple, cored

2 oz of coconut water

Preparation:

Combine blackberries and strawberries in a colander. Wash under cold running water and set aside.

Wash the grapes and set aside.

Wash the apple and remove the core. Cut into bite-sized pieces and set aside.

Now, process blackberries, grapes, strawberries, and apple in a juicer. Transfer to serving glasses and stir in the coconut water.

Add some ice cubes before serving.

Nutritional information per serving: Kcal: 201, Protein: 4.3g, Carbs: 63.4g, Fats: 1.7g

13. Carrot Apple Juice

Ingredients:

2 large carrots

1 large Granny Smith Apple

2 cups of butternut squash, seeded

1 small ginger root slice

Preparation:

Wash the carrots and cut into thick slices. Set aside.

Wash the apple and remove the core. Cut into bite-sized pieces and set aside.

Peel the butternut squash and remove the seeds using a spoon. Cut into small cubes and fill the measuring cup. Reserve the rest of the squash for some other juice. Wrap in a plastic foil and refrigerate.

Peel the ginger slice and set aside.

Now, process carrots, apple, butternut squash, and ginger in a juicer.

Transfer to serving glasses and refrigerate before serving.

Nutrition information per serving: Kcal: 246, Protein: 5.1g, Carbs: 75g, Fats: 1.1g

14.   Garlic Asparagus Juice

Ingredients:

2 medium-sized zucchinis, peeled and chopped

1 garlic clove, peeled

6 asparagus stalks, trimmed

3 Roma tomatoes, chopped

4 large carrots

¼ tsp salt

Preparation:

Peel the garlic clove and set aside.

Wash the asparagus and remove the woody ends. Chop into small pieces and set aside.

Peel the zucchinis and remove the seeds. Cut into bite-sized chunks and set aside.

Wash the tomatoes and cut into quarters. Cut in a bowl to reserve the juices. Set aside.

Wash the carrots and cut into small pieces. Set aside.

Combine garlic, asparagus, tomatoes, zucchinis, and carrots in a juicer and process until juiced.

Transfer to serving glasses and add a little bit of water to adjust the thickness of the juice.

Serve immediately.

Nutritional information per serving: Kcal: 92, Protein: 5.4g, Carbs: 27.3g, Fats: 0.9g

15.   Broccoli Mustard Green Juice

Ingredients:

1 cup of fresh broccoli

1 cup of mustard greens, torn

2 large artichokes, peeled and chopped

1 cup of fresh basil, torn

1 large cucumber

3-4 spinach leaves, torn

¼ tsp of Cayenne pepper, ground

Preparation:

Wash the broccoli and cut into small pieces. Set aside.

Combine mustard greens, basil, and spinach in a colander. Wash under cold running water and torn with hands. Set aside.

Trim off the outer leaves of artichokes using a sharp knife. Cut into small pieces and set aside.

Wash the cucumber and cut into thick slices. Set aside.

Now, process broccoli, mustard greens, artichokes, basil, spinach, and cucumber in a juicer.

Transfer to serving glasses and stir in the Cayenne pepper. You can add some salt, but this is optional.

Refrigerate for 5 minutes before serving.

Nutritional information per serving: Kcal: 157, Protein: 18.3g, Carbs: 55.4g, Fats: 1.6g

16.   Apricot Collard Green Juice

Ingredients:

1 whole apricot, cored

1 cup of collard greens, torn

2 small golden delicious apples, peeled and cored

¼ cup of pure coconut water, unsweetened

1 basil leaf

Preparation:

Wash the apricot and cut in half. Remove the pit and cut into small pieces. Set aside.

Wash the collard greens thoroughly and torn with hands. Set aside.

Wash and peel the apples. Remove the core and cut into bite-sized pieces. Set aside.

Now, process apricot, collard greens, and apples in a juicer. Process until juiced. Transfer to serving glasses and stir in the coconut water.

Garnish with basil leaf and add some ice before serving.

Enjoy!

Nutritional information per serving: Kcal: 144, Protein: 2.3g, Carbs: 44.9g, Fats: 0.9g

17.   Mint Apple Juice

Ingredients:

1 cup of fresh mint, torn

2 medium-sized red apples, cored

1 cup of fresh strawberries

1 large honeydew melon wedge

2 oz of coconut water

Preparation:

Wash the mint thoroughly and torn with hands. Set aside.

Wash the apples and remove the core. Cut into bite-sized pieces. Set aside.

Wash the strawberries under cold running water and cut in small pieces. Set aside.

Cut the honeydew melon lengthwise in half. Scoop out the seeds using a spoon. Cut the large wedges and peel them. Cut into small chunks and place in a bowl. Wrap the rest of the melon in a plastic foil and refrigerate. Now, process mint, apples, strawberries, and honeydew melon in a juicer. Transfer to serving glasses and stir in the coconut water. Add ice cubes and serve immediately.

Nutritional information per serving: Kcal: 293, Protein: 4.5g, Carbs: 84g, Fats: 1.6g

18.   Cucumber Cantaloupe Juice

Ingredients:

1 large cucumber, sliced

1 cup of cantaloupe, peeled and cubed

1 large mango, chunked

2 tbsp of fresh mint

Preparation:

Wash the cucumber and cut into thick slices. Set aside.

Cut the cantaloupe in half. Scoop out the seeds and flesh. Cut two wedges and peel them. Chop into chunks and set aside. Reserve the rest of the cantaloupe in a refrigerator.

Wash the mango and cut into bite-sized pieces. Set aside.

Now, process cucumber, cantaloupe, and mango in a juicer.

Transfer to serving glasses and add few ice cubes before serving.

Garnish with mint leaves and enjoy!

Nutrition information per serving: Kcal: 268, Protein: 6.1g, Carbs: 74.4g, Fats: 1.9g

19.   Cabbage Cucumber Juice

Ingredients:

1 cup of purple cabbage, torn

1 whole cucumber

5 large plums, pitted and halved

1 large lemon, peeled

1 cup of beets, trimmed

2 oz of water

Preparation:

Wash the cabbage thoroughly under cold running water. Drain and torn with hands.

Wash the cucumber and cut into thick slices. Set aside.

Wash the plums and cut in half. Remove the pits and cut into quarters. Set aside. Peel the lemon and cut lengthwise in half. Set aside. Wash the beets and trim off the green parts. Cut into bite-sized pieces and set aside. Now, process cabbage, cucumber, plums, lemon, and beets in a juicer. Transfer to serving glasses and add some ice before serving.

Nutrition information per serving: Kcal: 243, Protein: 8.3g, Carbs: 73.6g, Fats: 1.7g

20.   Celery Leek Juice

Ingredients:

1 cup of fresh celery

3 large leek

2 cups of beet greens, trimmed

1 small yellow onion slice

1 cup of fresh kale

1 large cucumber

1 ginger knob, sliced

½ tsp of Himalayan salt

Preparation:

Wash the celery and leek. Cut into small pieces and set aside.

Wash the beet greens and kale thoroughly and torn with hands. Set aside.

Peel the onion and cut in half. Cut one slice and reserve the rest for some other juice or meal.

Wash the cucumber and cut into thick slices. Set aside.

Peel the ginger and set aside.

Now, process celery, leek, beet greens, kale, onion, cucumber, and ginger in a juicer.

Transfer to serving glasses and stir in the salt.

Refrigerate for 10 minutes before serving.

Nutritional information per serving: Kcal: 230, Protein: 11.5g, Carbs: 63.2g, Fats: 2.1g

21. Pineapple Cherry Juice

Ingredients:

1 large Granny Smith apple, cored

1 cup of pineapple chunks

1 cup of cherries, pitted

2 large kiwis, peeled

Preparation:

Cut the top of a pineapple and peel it using a sharp knife. Cut into small chunks. Reserve the rest of the pineapple in a refrigerator.

Wash the cherries under cold running water. Drain and remove the pits. Set aside.

Wash the apple and remove the core. Cut into bite-sized pieces and set aside.

Peel the kiwis and cut lengthwise in half. Set aside.

Now, combine pineapple, cherries, apple, and kiwis in a juicer and process until juiced.

Transfer to serving glasses and serve immediately.

Nutrition information per serving: Kcal: 287, Protein: 4.2g, Carbs: 84.5g, Fats: 1.2g

22.   Zucchini Potato Juice

Ingredients:

1 large zucchini, seeded

1 cup of sweet potatoes, chopped

1 cup of parsnips, chopped

1 ginger root slice, 1-inch

2 oz of water

Preparation:

Peel the zucchini and cut in half. Scrape out the seeds with a spoon. Cut into chunks and set aside.

Peel the sweet potato and cut into chunks. Fill the measuring cup and reserve the rest for some other juice. Set aside.

Wash the parsnips and trim off the green parts. Cut into thick slices and fill the measuring cup. Reserve the rest for some other juice. Peel the ginger root and set aside.

Now, process zucchini, sweet potato, parsnips, and ginger in a juicer. Transfer to serving glasses and stir in the water.

Refrigerate for 5 minutes before serving.

Nutrition information per serving: Kcal: 216, Protein: 7.6g, Carbs: 61.1g, Fats: 1.5g

23. Lettuce Squash Juice

Ingredients:

1 cup of Romaine lettuce, torn

1 cup of red leaf lettuce, torn

1 cup of butternut squash, cubed

1 cup of celery, chopped

1 cup of mustard greens, torn

1 cup of Brussels sprouts, halved

1 large lemon, peeled

1 large cucumber

Preparation:

Combine mustard greens, Romaine lettuce, and red leaf lettuce in a colander and wash under cold running water. Drain and torn with hands. Set aside.

Peel the butternut squash and remove the seeds using a spoon. Cut into small cubes and reserve the rest of the squash for some other recipe. Wrap in a plastic foil and refrigerate.

Wash the celery and cut into small pieces. Set aside.

Wash the Brussels sprouts and trim off the outer leaves.

Cut in half and set aside.

Peel the lemon and cut lengthwise in half. Set aside.

Wash the cucumber and cut into thick slices. Set aside.

Now, process celery, mustard greens, Romaine lettuce, red leaf lettuce, squash, Brussel sprouts, lemon, and cucumber in a juicer.

Transfer to serving glasses and add some ice before serving.

Enjoy!

Nutrition information per serving: Kcal: 152, Protein: 10.2g, Carbs: 48.4g, Fats: 1.5g

24.   Lime Celery Juice

Ingredients:

1 large lime, peeled

5 small celery stalks

¼ cup of fresh mint

¼ cup of fresh spinach

3oz of coconut water

Preparation:

Peel the lime and cut into quarters. Set aside.

Wash the celery stalks and chop into small pieces. Set aside.

Wash the spinach and mint in a colander. Chop and place in a medium bowl. Add lukewarm water and let it stand for 5 minutes.

Now, combine lime, celery, mint, and spinach in a juicer and process until juiced.

Transfer to serving glasses and stir in the coconut water.

Refrigerate for 5 minutes and serve!

Nutritional information per serving: Kcal: 45, Protein: 2.2g, Carbs: 16.8g, Fats: 1.6g

25.   Pepper Apple Juice

Ingredients:

1 large red bell pepper, seeded

1 large red apple, cored

5 large radishes, trimmed

1 cup of red leaf lettuce

1 large lemon, peeled

1 cup of watercress

½ tsp of Himalayan salt

Preparation:

Wash the pepper and cut in half. Remove the seeds and cut into small pieces. Set aside.

Wash the apple and remove the core. Cut into bite-sized pieces and set aside.

Wash the radishes and trim off the green parts. Cut in half and set aside.

Combine red leaf lettuce and watercress in a colander and wash under cold running water. Torn with hands and set aside.

Peel the lemon and cut lengthwise in half. Set aside.

Now, process pepper, apple, radishes, red leaf lettuce, watercress, and lemon in a juicer.

Transfer to serving glasses stir in the Himalayan salt.

Add few ice cubes before serving.

Nutrition information per serving: Kcal: 352, Protein: 7.6g, Carbs: 41.6g, Fats: 30.3g

26.   Watermelon Orange Juice

Ingredients:

2 cups of watermelon, seeded

1 large orange, peeled

1 cup of fresh basil, chopped

1 cup of Romaine lettuce, chopped

¼ tsp of jalapeno pepper, ground

Preparation:

Cut the watermelon lengthwise. For two cups, you will need about two large wedges. Peel and cut into chunks. Remove the seeds and set aside. Reserve the rest of the melon for some other juices.

Peel the orange and divide into wedges. Set aside.

Combine lettuce and basil in a colander and wash under cold running water. Drain and chop into small pieces. Set aside. Now, process watermelon, orange, lettuce, and basil in a juicer. Process until juiced. Transfer to serving glasses and stir in the jalapeno pepper for some extra spicy flavor.

Refrigerate for 5 minutes before serving.

Enjoy!

Nutrition information per serving: Kcal: 165, Protein: 4.9g, Carbs: 46.7g, Fats: 1g

27.   Apple Cucumber Juice

Ingredients:

1 medium-sized apple, cored

1 large cucumber, sliced

1 cup of yellow pumpkin, cubed

1 knob of ginger root, sliced

2 large carrots

¼ tsp of cinnamon, ground

Preparation:

Wash the apple and remove the core. Cut into bite-sized pieces and set aside.

Wash the cucumber and carrots and cut into thick slices. Set aside.ž

Peel the pumpkin and cut in half. Scoop out the seeds using a spoon. Cut one large wedge and peel it. Cut into small chunks and set aside. Reserve the rest for later. Peel the ginger knob and chop into small pieces. Set aside. Now, process pumpkin, ginger, apple, and cucumber in a juicer. Transfer to serving glasses and stir in the cinnamon.

Add some ice and serve immediately.

Nutrition information per serving: Kcal: 194, Protein: 5.3g, Carbs: 56.1g, Fats: 1.4g

28.   Kale Lettuce Juice

Ingredients:

1 cup of kale, chopped

1 cup of Romaine lettuce, chopped

1 cup of turnip greens, chopped

1 cup of cauliflower, chopped

1 large cucumber, sliced

Preparation:

Combine kale, turnip greens, and Romaine lettuce in a colander and wash under cold running water. Drain and roughly chop it. Set aside.

Trim off the outer leaves of cauliflower. Wash it and cut into small pieces. Fill the measuring cup and reserve the rest for some other juice. Set aside. Wash the cucumber and cut into thick slices. Set aside.

Now, combine kale, Romaine lettuce, turnip greens, cauliflower, and cucumber in a juicer and process until juiced. Transfer to serving glasses and add some ice before serving.

Enjoy!

Nutrition information per serving: Kcal: 96, Protein: 8.3g, Carbs: 27.6g, Fats: 1.6g

29.   Fennel Pepper Juice

Ingredients:

1 large fennel bulb

1 large bell pepper, seeded

1 large yellow apple, cored

1 cup of fresh kale, chopped

1 cup of mustard greens

Preparation:

Wash the fennel bulb and trim off the wilted outer layers. Cut into small chunks and set aside.

Wash the bell pepper and cut in half. Remove the seeds and chop into small slices. Set aside.

Wash the apple and remove the core. Cut into bite-sized pieces and set aside.

Combine kale and mustard greens in a colander. Wash under cold running water and torn with hands. Set aside.

Now, process fennel, bell pepper, apple, kale, mustard greens in a juicer. Transfer to serving glasses and refrigerate for 5 minutes before serving.

Nutrition information per serving: Kcal: 199, Protein: 9.4g, Carbs: 62.4g, Fats: 1.9g

30.   Carrot Lime Juice

Ingredients:

2 large carrots, sliced

1 large lime, peeled

1 cup of pineapple chunks

1 large Granny Smith apple, cored

¼ tsp of red pepper, ground

Preparation:

Wash the carrots and chop into thick slices. Set aside.

Peel the lime and cut lengthwise in half. Set aside.

Cut the top of a pineapple and peel it using a sharp knife. Cut into small chunks. Reserve the rest of the pineapple in a refrigerator.

Wash the apple and remove the core. Cut into bite-sized pieces and set aside.

Now, combine carrots, lime, pineapple, and apple in a juicer and process until juiced. Transfer to serving glasses and stir in the red pepper. Add some water to adjust the thickness of the juice. However, this is optional. Refrigerate for 5 minutes before serving.

Nutrition information per serving: Kcal: 224, Protein: 3.3g, Carbs: 67.1g, Fats: 1.1g

31.   Lemon Carrot Juice

Ingredients:

1 large lemon, peeled

1 large carrot, sliced

1 cup of apricots, pitted and halved

1 medium-sized green apple, cored

1 tbsp of liquid honey

2 oz of water

Preparation:

Peel the lemon and cut lengthwise in half. Set aside.

Wash the carrot and cut into thick slices and set aside.

Wash the apricots and cut in half. Remove the pits and fill the measuring cup. Reserve the rest for some other juice. Set aside.

Wash the apple and remove the core. Cut into bite-sized pieces and set aside. Now, combine lemon, carrot, apricots, and apple in a juicer and process until juiced. Transfer to serving glasses and stir in the liquid honey and water.

Refrigerate for 10 minutes before serving.

Nutrition information per serving: Kcal: 243, Protein: 4.2g, Carbs: 69.3g, Fats: 1.3g

32.   Cucumber Celery Juice

Ingredients:

1 large cucumber

4-5 medium celery stalks

2 large oranges, peeled

1 cup of Swiss chards, torn

1 small lemon, peeled

A handful of parsley, torn

Preparation:

Wash the cucumber and cut into thick slices. Set aside.

Wash the celery stalks and chop into small pieces. Set aside. Peel the oranges and divide into wedges. Set aside.

Combine Swiss chards and parsley in a colander and wash thoroughly under cold running water. Drain and torn with hands. Set aside. Peel the lemon and cut lengthwise in half. Set aside.

Now, process cucumber, celery, oranges, Swiss chards, parsley, and lemon in a juicer. Transfer to serving glasses and refrigerate for 10 minutes before serving.

Nutrition information per serving: Kcal: 214, Protein: 8.4g, Carbs: 67.6g, Fats: 1.5g

33.   Pear Broccoli Juice

Ingredients:

1 large pear, cored

1 cup of fresh broccoli, chopped

1 medium-sized zucchini

1 large fennel bulb

1 small ginger root slice

Preparation:

Wash the pear and remove the core. Cut into small pieces and set aside.

Wash the broccoli and cut into small pieces and set aside.

Peel the zucchini and cut in half. Scrape out the seeds with a spoon. Cut into chunks and set aside.

Trim off the outer leaves of the artichoke using a sharp knife. Cut into small pieces and set aside.

Peel the ginger root and set aside. Now, process pear, broccoli, zucchini, fennel, and ginger in a juicer. Transfer to serving glasses and add some ice before serving.

Nutrition information per serving: Kcal: 195, Protein: 8.7g, Carbs: 64.5g, Fats: 1.8g

34.   Carrot Lemon Juice

Ingredients:

3 large carrots

1 large lemon, peeled

2 large beets, trimmed

1 medium-sized green apple, cored

3-4 large celery stalks

¼ tsp of ginger, ground

A handful of fresh kale, torn

Preparation:

Wash the carrots and cut into thick slices. Set aside.

Peel the lemon and cut lengthwise in half. Set aside.

Wash the beets and trim off the green parts. Cut into bite-sized pieces and set aside.

Wash the apple and remove the core. Cut into bite-sized pieces and set aside.

Wash the celery stalks and chop into small pieces. Set aside.

Wash the kale thoroughly and torn with hands. Set aside.

Now, process carrots, lemon, beets, apple, celery, and kale in a juicer.

Transfer to serving glasses and stir in the ginger. Add some ice and serve immediately.

Nutrition information per serving: Kcal: 136, Protein: 6.1g, Carbs: 39g, Fats: 1.2g

35. Raspberry Apple Juice

Ingredients:

1 cup of raspberries

1 medium-sized apple, cored

1 large grapefruit, peeled

1 large carrot

1 small ginger root slice, 1-inch

1 oz of water

Preparation:

Place the raspberries in a colander and wash under cold running water. Drain and set aside.

Wash the apple and remove the core. Cut into bite-sized pieces. Set aside.

Peel the grapefruit and divide into wedges. Set aside.

Wash the carrot and cut into thick slices. Set aside. Peel the ginger root and set aside.

Now, process raspberries, apple, carrot, grapefruit, and ginger in a juicer. Transfer to serving glasses and stir in the water. Add few ice cubes or refrigerate before serving.

Nutrition information per serving: Kcal: 239, Protein: 4.9g, Carbs: 76.2g, Fats: 1.7g

36.   Beet Kale Juice

Ingredients:

1 large beet, trimmed

1 cup of purple kale, torn

1 cup of red leaf lettuce, torn

2 large carrots, sliced

1 large lemon, peeled

¼ tsp of ginger, ground

Preparation:

Combine red leaf lettuce and kale in a colander. Wash under cold running water and drain. Torn with hands and set aside.

Wash the beet and trim off the green parts. Cut into small pieces and set aside.

Wash the carrots and cut into thick slices. Set aside. Peel the lemon and cut lengthwise in half. Set aside. Now, combine beet, kale, lettuce, carrots, and lemon in a juicer and process until juiced. Transfer to serving glasses and add some ice before serving.

Nutrition information per serving: Kcal: 135, Protein: 7.9g, Carbs: 41.7g, Fats: 1.5g

37.   Asparagus Celery Juice

Ingredients:

1 cup of asparagus, trimmed

1 cup of fresh celery

1 cup of green beans

1 large cucumber

1 cup of Romaine lettuce

1 large apple, cored

1 oz of water

Preparation:

Wash the asparagus and trim off the woody ends. Cut into small pieces and set aside.

Wash the celery and cut into bite-sized pieces. Set aside.

Wash the green beans and cut into 1-inch pieces. Set aside.

Wash the cucumber and cut into thick slices. Set aside.

Wash the lettuce thoroughly under cold running water. Drain and torn with hands. Set aside.

Wash the apple and remove the core. Cut into bite-sized pieces and set aside.

Now, process asparagus, celery, green beans, cucumber, lettuce and apple in a juicer. Transfer to serving glasses and stir in some water.

Add some ice and serve.

Nutrition information per serving: Kcal: 185, Protein: 8.1g, Carbs: 52.5g, Fats: 1.3g

38.   Blueberry Apple Juice

Ingredients:

1 cup of blueberries

1 medium-sized apple, cored

1 cup of beets, trimmed

2 small carrots, sliced

1 large lemon, peeled

2 oz of coconut water

A few mint leaves

Preparation:

Wash the blueberries under cold running water. Drain and set aside.

Wash the apple and remove the core. Cut into small pieces and set aside.

Wash the beets and trim off the green parts. Cut into bite-sized pieces and set aside.

Wash the carrots and cut into thick slices. Set aside.

Peel the lemon and cut lengthwise in half. Set aside.

Now, process blueberries, apple, beets, carrots, and lemon

in a juicer.

Transfer to serving glasses and stir in the coconut water. Garnish with mint and refrigerate before serving.

Enjoy!

Nutrition information per serving: Kcal: 240, Protein: 5.6g, Carbs: 74.1g, Fats: 1.5g

39. Cucumber Strawberry Juice

Ingredients:

1 large cucumber, sliced

1 cup of fresh strawberries, chopped

2 whole kiwis, peeled

1 small lime, peeled

2 tbsp of fresh mint

Preparation:

Wash the cucumber and chop into bite-sized pieces.

Wash the strawberries and cut into halves. Set aside.

Peel the kiwis and cut into halves. Set aside.

Peel the lime and cut into quarters. Set aside.

Wash the mint leaves and soak in water for 5 minutes.

Now, combine cucumber, strawberries, kiwis, lime, and mint in a juicer. Process until nicely juiced.

Transfer to serving glasses and refrigerate for 5 minutes before serving.

Nutritional information per serving: Kcal: 91, Protein: 3.1g, Carbs: 29.9g, Fats: 0.9g

40.   Lemon Lime Juice

Ingredients:

1 large lemon, peeled

1 large lime, peeled

1 large cucumber

1 large orange, peeled

1 tbsp of chia seeds

2 oz of water

Preparation:

Peel the lemon and lime and cut lengthwise in half. Set aside.

Wash the cucumber and cut into thick slices. Set aside.

Peel the orange and divide into wedges. Set aside.

Now, combine lemon, lime, cucumber, and orange in a juicer and process until juiced. Transfer to serving glasses and stir in some chia seeds for some extra nutrients.

Add few ice cubes and refrigerate for 5 minutes before serving.

Stir in the water after refrigerating and enjoy!

Nutrition information per serving: Kcal: 186, Protein: 6.2g, Carbs: 41.4g, Fats: 5g

41.   Lemon Pepper Juice

Ingredients:

1 large lemon, peeled

1 large bell pepper, seeded

1 large red apple, cored

3 tbsp of chia seeds

Preparation:

Peel the lemon and cut into quarters. Set aside.

Wash the bell pepper and cut into halves. Remove the seeds and then chop into small pieces.

Wash the apple and remove the core. Cut into bite-sized pieces and set aside.

Now, combine lemon, bell pepper, and apple in a juicer. Process until juiced.

Transfer to serving glasses and stir in the chia seeds. Add a little bit of water because chia will soak up the liquid.

Stir well and refrigerate for about 10 minutes.

Enjoy!

Nutritional information per serving: Kcal: 135, Protein: 4.2g, Carbs: 31.3g, Fats: 6.2g

42. Pineapple Cucumber Juice

Ingredients:

1 cup of pineapple chunks

1 large cucumber, sliced

1 large grapefruit, peeled

1 small apple, cored

1 small ginger root slice, finely chopped

1 large lemon, peeled

Preparation:

Cut the top of a pineapple and peel it using a sharp knife. Cut into small chunks. Reserve the rest of the pineapple in a refrigerator.

Peel the grapefruit and divide into wedges. Set aside.

Wash the cucumber and cut into thick slices. Set aside.

Wash the apple and remove the core. Cut into bite-sized pieces and set aside.

Peel the ginger root slice and set aside.

Peel the lemon and cut lengthwise in half. Set aside.

Now, process pineapple, cucumber, grapefruit, apple,

ginger, and lemon in a juicer.

Transfer to serving glasses and refrigerate for 10 minutes before serving.

Enjoy!

Nutrition information per serving: Kcal: 280, Protein: 6.1g, Carbs: 84.2g, Fats: 1.3g

43.   Carrot Lime Juice

Ingredients:

2 large carrots

1 large lime, peeled

1 large papaya, seeded and peeled

2 oz of coconut water

Preparation:

Wash the carrots and cut into thick slices. Set aside.

Peel the lime and cut lengthwise in half. Set aside.

Peel the papaya and cut lengthwise in half. Scoop out the black seeds and flesh using a spoon. Cut into small chunks. Set aside.

Now, combine carrots, lime, and papaya in a juicer and process until juiced.

Transfer to serving glasses and stir in the coconut water.

Add few ice cubes or refrigerate before serving.

Nutrition information per serving: Kcal: 347, Protein: 5.2g, Carbs: 119g, Fats: 2.4g

44.   Cantaloupe Radish Juice

Ingredients:

1 cup of cantaloupe, cubed

2 medium-sized radishes, trimmed

2 large oranges, peeled

1 ginger root knob, 1-inch

1 tbsp of liquid honey

2 oz of water

Preparation:

Cut the cantaloupe in half. Scoop out the seeds and flesh. You will need about one large wedge for one cup. Cut and peel it. Chop into chunks and set aside. Reserve the rest of the cantaloupe in a refrigerator.

Wash the radishes and trim off the green parts. Cut into small pieces and set aside. Peel the oranges and divide into wedges. Set aside. Peel the ginger root knob and set aside. Now, process oranges, cantaloupe, radishes, and ginger in a juicer. Transfer to serving glasses and stir in the honey and water. Add few ice cubes or refrigerate for 5 minutes before serving.

Nutrition information per serving: Kcal: 250, Protein: 4.9g, Carbs: 74.3g, Fats: 0.8g

45.   Asparagus Kale Juice

Ingredients:

1 cup of fresh asparagus, trimmed

1 cup of fresh kale, torn

1 large artichoke head

1 large Roma tomato, chopped

3 tbsp of fresh parsley, roughly chopped

Preparation:

Wash the asparagus and trim off the woody ends. Cut into small pieces and set aside.

Wash the kale and parsley thoroughly and torn with hands. Set aside.

Trim off the outer leaves of the artichoke using a sharp knife. Cut into small pieces and set aside.

Wash the tomato and place in a bowl. Cut into small pieces and reserve the juice.

Now, process asparagus, kale, artichoke, tomato, and parsley in a juicer. Add the reserved tomato juice.

Transfer to serving glasses and refrigerate for 10 minutes.

Nutrition information per serving: Kcal: 107, Protein: 13.1g, Carbs: 35.9g, Fats: 1.5g

46.   Apple Tangerine Juice

Ingredients:

1 large green apple, cored

4 tangerines, peeled

1 large fennel

½ cup of fresh kale

Preparation:

Wash and core the apple. Cut into bite-sized pieces and set aside.

Peel the tangerines and divide into wedges. Set aside.

Trim off the fennel stalks and wilted outer layers. Cut into bite-sized pieces and set aside.

Wash the kale thoroughly and roughly chop it. Set aside.

Now, combine apple, tangerines, fennel, and kale in a juicer. Process until nicely juiced. Transfer to a serving glass and add some ice.

Serve immediately.

Nutritional information per serving: Kcal: 121, Protein: 4.3g, Carbs: 31.3g, Fats: 1.3g

47.   Avocado Cucumber Juice

Ingredients:

1 large artichoke heart

1 cup of avocado, cubed

1 large cucumber

1 cup of fresh basil

1 cup of green cabbage

1 tbsp of liquid honey

Preparation:

Peel the avocado and cut in half. Remove the pit and cut into cubes. Reserve the rest of the avocado for some other juice. Set aside.

Wash the cucumber and cut into thick slices. Set aside.

Using a sharp knife, trim off the outer leaves of the artichoke. Wash it and cut into small pieces. Set aside.

Wash the basil and cabbage thoroughly and torn with hands. Set aside. Now, process avocado, cucumber, artichoke, basil, and cabbage in a juicer. Transfer to serving glasses and stir in the liquid honey. Refrigerate for 5 minutes before serving.

Nutrition information per serving: Kcal: 357, Protein: 12.1g, Carbs: 63.6g, Fats: 22.8g

48.   Plum Cucumber Juice

Ingredients:

1 cup of fresh plums, pitted

1 large cucumber, sliced

2 cups of green grapes

1 cup of mustard greens, torn

1 small ginger root slice, 1-inch

Preparation:

Wash the plums and cut in half. Remove the pits and set aside.

Wash the cucumber and cut into thick slices. Set aside.

Wash the grapes under cold running water. Drain and set aside.

Wash the mustard greens thoroughly and torn with hands. Set aside. Peel the ginger root slice and set aside.

Now, process plums, cucumber, grapes, mustard greens, and ginger in a juicer. Transfer to serving glasses and refrigerate for 5 minutes before serving.

Enjoy!

Nutrition information per serving: Kcal: 339, Protein: 6.9g, Carbs: 56.7g, Fats: 21.9g

ADDITIONAL TITLES FROM THIS AUTHOR

70 Effective Meal Recipes to Prevent and Solve Being Overweight: Burn Fat Fast by Using Proper Dieting and Smart Nutrition

By

Joe Correa CSN

48 Acne Solving Meal Recipes: The Fast and Natural Path to Fixing Your Acne Problems in Less Than 10 Days!

By

Joe Correa CSN

41 Alzheimer's Preventing Meal Recipes: Reduce or Eliminate Your Alzheimer's Condition in 30 Days or Less!

By

Joe Correa CSN

70 Effective Breast Cancer Meal Recipes: Prevent and Fight Breast Cancer with Smart Nutrition and Powerful Foods

By

Joe Correa CSN

www.ingramcontent.com/pod-product-compliance
Lightning Source LLC
Chambersburg PA
CBHW030249030426
42336CB00009B/310